Recipe:

Rating: ☆☆☆☆☆ Difficulty: ☆☆☆☆☆ Prep Time: Cook Time:

Ingredients:

Cooking Instructions:

Thoughts and Notes:

Recipe:

Rating: ☆☆☆☆☆ Difficulty: ✿✿✿✿✿ Prep Time: Cook Time:

Ingredients:
_____
_____
_____
_____
_____
_____
_____

Cooking Instructions:
_____
_____
_____
_____
_____
_____
_____
_____
_____
_____
_____
_____

Thoughts and Notes:
_____
_____
_____
_____
_____
_____

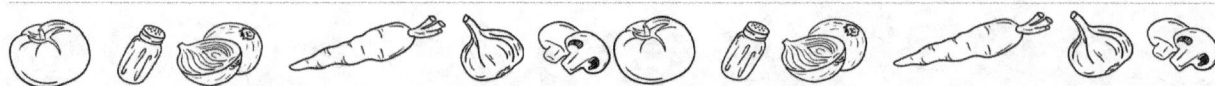

Recipe:

Rating: ☆☆☆☆☆ Difficulty: ☆☆☆☆☆ Prep Time:　　　　Cook Time:

Ingredients:

Cooking Instructions:

Thoughts and Notes:

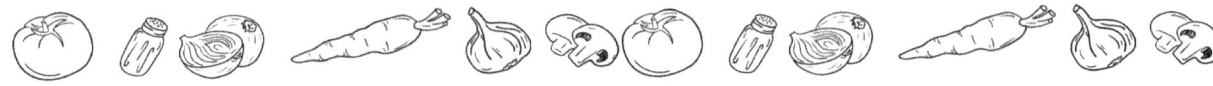

Recipe:

Rating: ☆☆☆☆☆ Difficulty: ☆☆☆☆☆ Prep Time: Cook Time:

Ingredients:

Cooking Instructions:

Thoughts and Notes:

Recipe:

Rating: ☆☆☆☆☆ Difficulty: ☆☆☆☆☆ Prep Time: Cook Time:

Ingredients:

Cooking Instructions:

Thoughts and Notes:

Recipe:

Rating: ☆☆☆☆☆ Difficulty: ✿✿✿✿✿ Prep Time: Cook Time:

Ingredients:
_____
_____
_____
_____
_____
_____

Cooking Instructions:
_____
_____
_____
_____
_____
_____
_____
_____
_____
_____

Thoughts and Notes:
_____
_____
_____
_____
_____

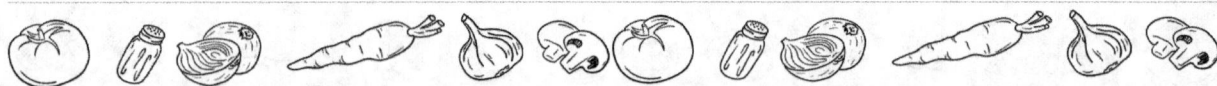

Recipe:

Rating: ☆☆☆☆☆ Difficulty: ☆☆☆☆☆ Prep Time: Cook Time:

Ingredients:

Cooking Instructions:

Thoughts and Notes:

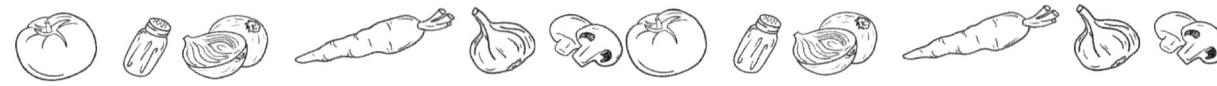

Recipe:

Rating: ☆☆☆☆ Difficulty: ☆☆☆☆ Prep Time: Cook Time:

Ingredients:

Cooking Instructions:

Thoughts and Notes:

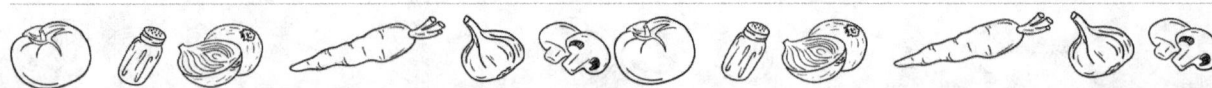

Recipe:

Rating: ☆☆☆☆☆ Difficulty: ☆☆☆☆☆ Prep Time: Cook Time:

Ingredients:

Cooking Instructions:

Thoughts and Notes:

Recipe:

Rating: ☆☆☆☆☆ Difficulty: ✿✿✿✿✿ Prep Time: Cook Time:

Ingredients:
_____
_____
_____
_____
_____
_____
_____

Cooking Instructions:
_____
_____
_____
_____
_____
_____
_____
_____
_____
_____
_____
_____

Thoughts and Notes:
_____
_____
_____
_____
_____

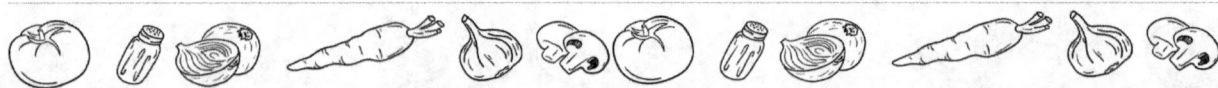

Recipe:

Rating: ☆☆☆☆☆ Difficulty: ☆☆☆☆☆ Prep Time: Cook Time:

Ingredients:

Cooking Instructions:

Thoughts and Notes:

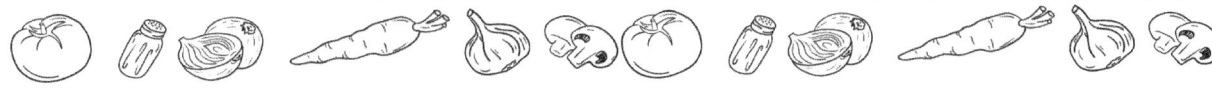

Recipe:

Rating: ☆☆☆☆☆ Difficulty: ☆☆☆☆☆ Prep Time: Cook Time:

Ingredients:

Cooking Instructions:

Thoughts and Notes:

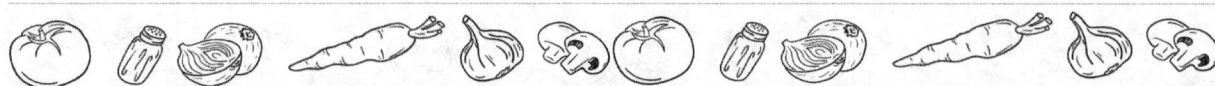

Recipe:

Rating: ☆☆☆☆☆ **Difficulty:** ☆☆☆☆☆ **Prep Time:**   **Cook Time:**

Ingredients:

Cooking Instructions:

Thoughts and Notes:

Recipe:

Rating: ☆☆☆☆☆ Difficulty: ✿✿✿✿✿ Prep Time: Cook Time:

Ingredients:

Cooking Instructions:

Thoughts and Notes:

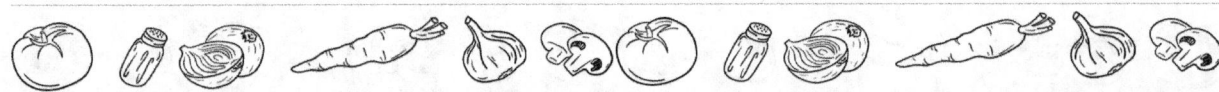

Recipe:

Rating: ☆☆☆☆☆ Difficulty: ☆☆☆☆☆ Prep Time: Cook Time:

Ingredients:

Cooking Instructions:

Thoughts and Notes:

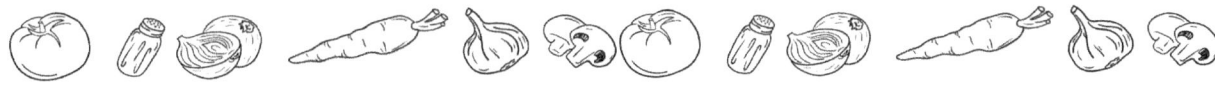

Recipe:

Rating: ☆☆☆☆☆ Difficulty: ☆☆☆☆☆ Prep Time: Cook Time:

Ingredients:

Cooking Instructions:

Thoughts and Notes:

Recipe:

Rating: ☆☆☆☆☆ Difficulty: ☆☆☆☆☆ Prep Time: Cook Time:

Ingredients:

Cooking Instructions:

Thoughts and Notes:

Recipe:

Rating: ☆☆☆☆☆ Difficulty: ✿✿✿✿✿ Prep Time: Cook Time:

Ingredients:
_____
_____
_____
_____
_____
_____

Cooking Instructions:
_____
_____
_____
_____
_____
_____
_____
_____
_____
_____
_____
_____

Thoughts and Notes:
_____
_____
_____
_____
_____

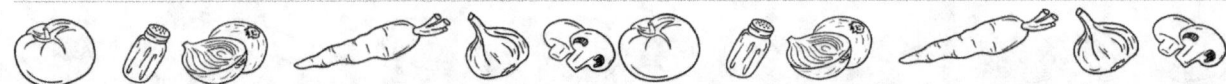

Recipe:

Rating: ☆☆☆☆☆ Difficulty: ☆☆☆☆☆ Prep Time: Cook Time:

Ingredients:

Cooking Instructions:

Thoughts and Notes:

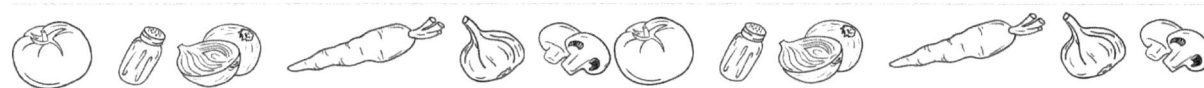

Recipe:

Rating: ☆☆☆☆☆ Difficulty: ☆☆☆☆☆ Prep Time: Cook Time:

Ingredients:

Cooking Instructions:

Thoughts and Notes:

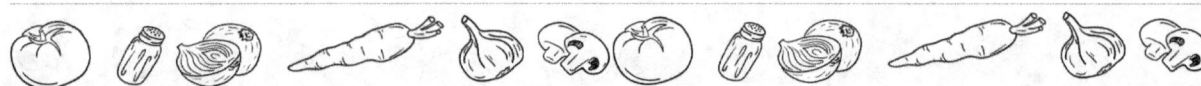

Recipe:

Rating: ☆☆☆☆☆ Difficulty: ☆☆☆☆☆ Prep Time: Cook Time:

Ingredients:

Cooking Instructions:

Thoughts and Notes:

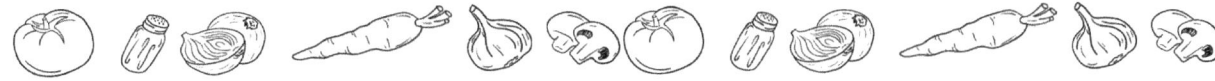

Recipe:

Rating: ☆☆☆☆☆ Difficulty: ✿✿✿✿✿ Prep Time: Cook Time:

Ingredients:

Cooking Instructions:

Thoughts and Notes:

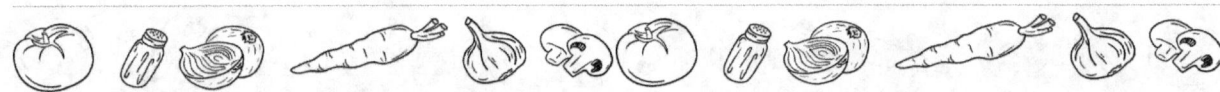

Recipe:

Rating: ☆☆☆☆☆ Difficulty: ☆☆☆☆☆ Prep Time: Cook Time:

Ingredients:

Cooking Instructions:

Thoughts and Notes:

Recipe:

Rating: ☆☆☆☆☆   Difficulty: ☆☆☆☆☆   Prep Time: Cook Time:

Ingredients:

Cooking Instructions:

Thoughts and Notes:

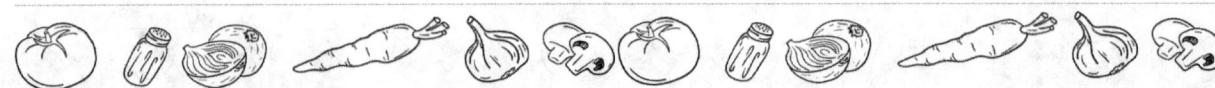

Recipe:

Rating: ☆☆☆☆☆ Difficulty: ☆☆☆☆☆ Prep Time: Cook Time:

Ingredients:

Cooking Instructions:

Thoughts and Notes:

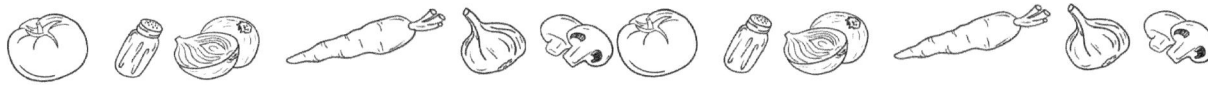

Recipe:

Rating: ☆☆☆☆☆ Difficulty: ☆☆☆☆☆ Prep Time: Cook Time:

Ingredients:

Cooking Instructions:

Thoughts and Notes:

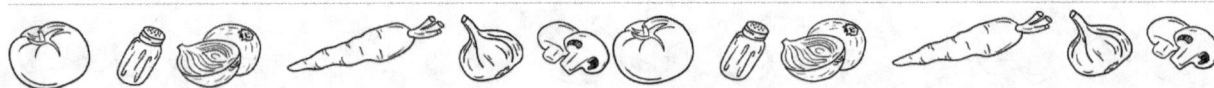

Recipe:

Rating: ☆☆☆☆☆ Difficulty: ☆☆☆☆☆ Prep Time: Cook Time:

Ingredients:

Cooking Instructions:

Thoughts and Notes:

Recipe:

Rating: ☆☆☆☆☆ Difficulty: ☆☆☆☆ Prep Time: Cook Time:

Ingredients:

Cooking Instructions:

Thoughts and Notes:

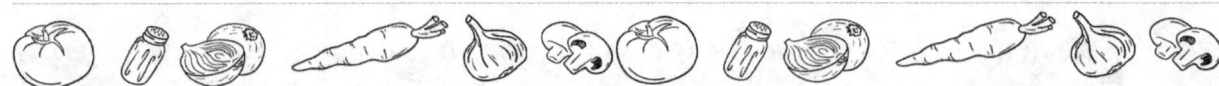

Recipe:

Rating: ☆☆☆☆☆ Difficulty: ☆☆☆☆☆ Prep Time: Cook Time:

Ingredients:

Cooking Instructions:

Thoughts and Notes:

Recipe:

Rating: ☆☆☆☆☆ Difficulty: ✿✿✿✿✿ Prep Time: Cook Time:

Ingredients:
_____
_____
_____
_____
_____
_____

Cooking Instructions:
_____
_____
_____
_____
_____
_____
_____
_____
_____
_____

Thoughts and Notes:
_____
_____
_____
_____

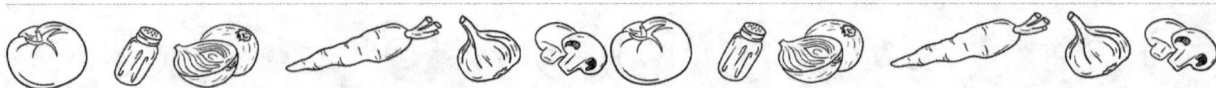

Recipe:

Rating: ☆☆☆☆☆ Difficulty: ☆☆☆☆☆ Prep Time: Cook Time:

Ingredients:

Cooking Instructions:

Thoughts and Notes:

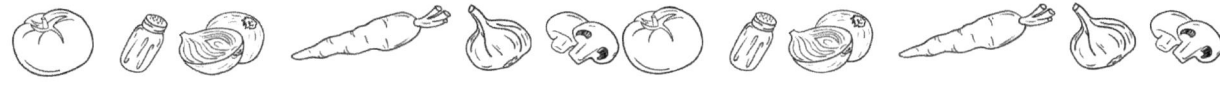

Recipe:

Rating: ☆☆☆☆☆ Difficulty: ✿✿✿✿✿ Prep Time: Cook Time:

Ingredients:

Cooking Instructions:

Thoughts and Notes:

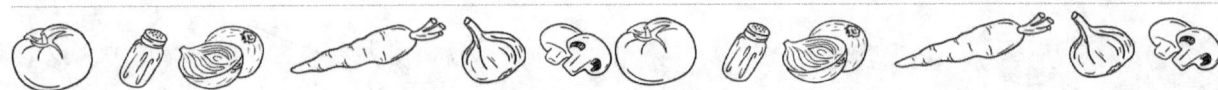

Recipe:

Rating: ☆☆☆☆☆ **Difficulty:** ☆☆☆☆☆ **Prep Time:**   **Cook Time:**

Ingredients:

Cooking Instructions:

Thoughts and Notes:

Recipe:

Rating: ☆☆☆☆☆ Difficulty: ❀❀❀❀❀ Prep Time: Cook Time:

Ingredients:

Cooking Instructions:

Thoughts and Notes:

Recipe:

Rating: ☆☆☆☆☆ Difficulty: ✿✿✿✿✿ Prep Time: Cook Time:

Ingredients:

Cooking Instructions:

Thoughts and Notes:

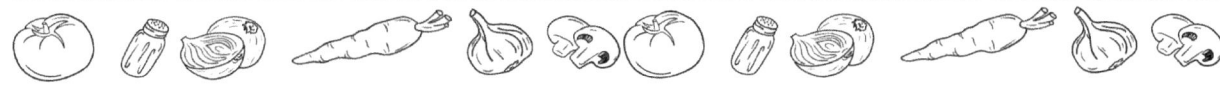

Recipe:

Rating: ☆☆☆☆☆   Difficulty: ☆☆☆☆☆   Prep Time: Cook Time:

Ingredients:

Cooking Instructions:

Thoughts and Notes:

Recipe:

Rating: ☆☆☆☆☆ Difficulty: ☆☆☆☆☆ Prep Time: Cook Time:

Ingredients:

Cooking Instructions:

Thoughts and Notes:

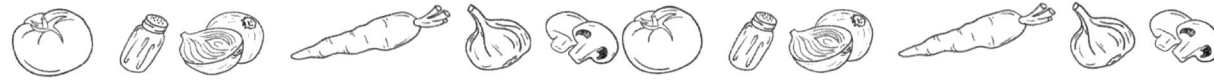

Recipe:

Rating: ☆☆☆☆ Difficulty: ☆☆☆☆ Prep Time: Cook Time:

Ingredients:

_____
_____
_____
_____
_____
_____

Cooking Instructions:

_____
_____
_____
_____
_____
_____
_____
_____
_____
_____

Thoughts and Notes:

_____
_____
_____
_____
_____
_____

Recipe:

Rating: ☆☆☆☆☆ Difficulty: ✿✿✿✿✿ Prep Time: Cook Time:

Ingredients:

Cooking Instructions:

Thoughts and Notes:

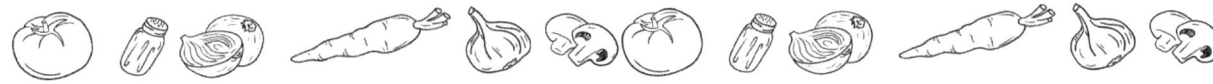

Recipe:

Rating: ☆☆☆☆☆ Difficulty: ☆☆☆☆☆ Prep Time: Cook Time:

Ingredients:

Cooking Instructions:

Thoughts and Notes:

Recipe:

Rating: ☆☆☆☆☆ Difficulty: ☆☆☆☆☆ Prep Time: Cook Time:

Ingredients:

Cooking Instructions:

Thoughts and Notes:

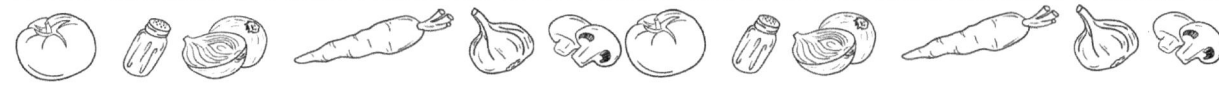

Recipe:

Rating: ☆☆☆☆☆ Difficulty: ✿✿✿✿✿ Prep Time: Cook Time:

Ingredients:

Cooking Instructions:

Thoughts and Notes:

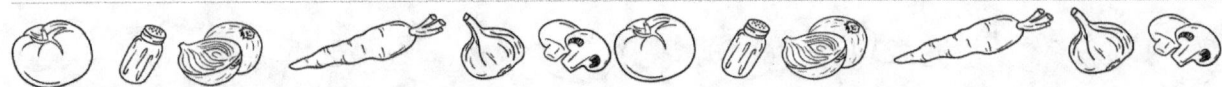

Recipe:

Rating: ☆☆☆☆☆ Difficulty: ☆☆☆☆☆ Prep Time: Cook Time:

Ingredients:

Cooking Instructions:

Thoughts and Notes:

Recipe:

Rating: ☆☆☆☆☆ Difficulty: ☆☆☆☆☆ Prep Time: Cook Time:

Ingredients:

Cooking Instructions:

Thoughts and Notes:

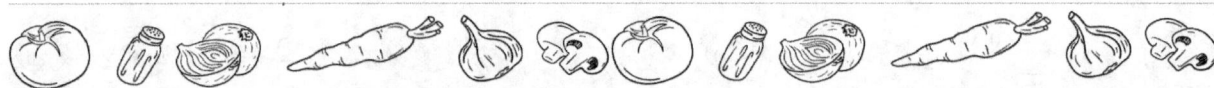

Recipe:

Rating: ☆☆☆☆☆   Difficulty: ☆☆☆☆☆   Prep Time: Cook Time:

Ingredients:

Cooking Instructions:

Thoughts and Notes:

Recipe:

Rating: ☆☆☆☆☆   Difficulty: ✿✿✿✿✿   Prep Time: Cook Time:

Ingredients:
_____
_____
_____
_____
_____
_____
_____

Cooking Instructions:
_____
_____
_____
_____
_____
_____
_____
_____
_____
_____
_____
_____

Thoughts and Notes:
_____
_____
_____
_____
_____

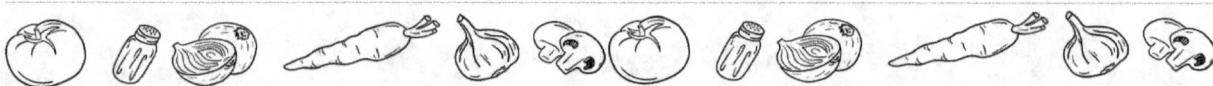

Recipe:

Rating: ☆☆☆☆☆ Difficulty: ☆☆☆☆☆ Prep Time: Cook Time:

Ingredients:

Cooking Instructions:

Thoughts and Notes:

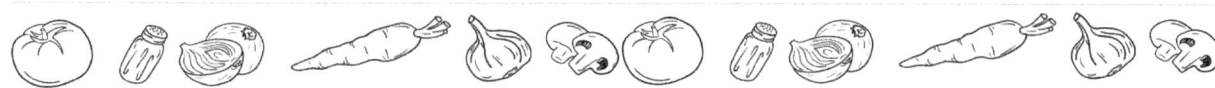

Recipe:

Rating: ☆☆☆☆☆ Difficulty: ☆☆☆☆☆ Prep Time: Cook Time:

Ingredients:

Cooking Instructions:

Thoughts and Notes:

Recipe:

Rating: ☆☆☆☆☆ Difficulty: ☆☆☆☆☆ Prep Time: Cook Time:

Ingredients:

Cooking Instructions:

Thoughts and Notes:

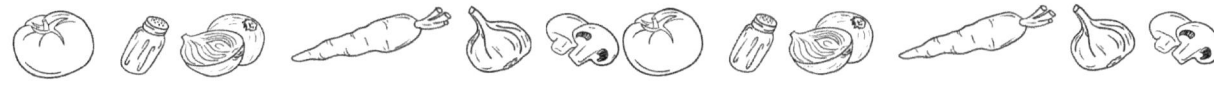

Recipe:

Rating: ☆☆☆☆☆   Difficulty: ☆☆☆☆   Prep Time: Cook Time:

Ingredients:

Cooking Instructions:

Thoughts and Notes:

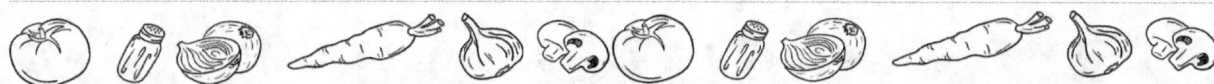

Recipe:

Rating: ☆☆☆☆☆ Difficulty: ✿✿✿✿✿ Prep Time: Cook Time:

Ingredients:

Cooking Instructions:

Thoughts and Notes:

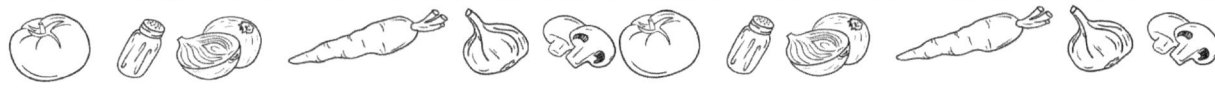

Recipe:

Rating: ☆☆☆☆☆   Difficulty: ☆☆☆☆☆   Prep Time: Cook Time:

Ingredients:
_____
_____
_____
_____
_____
_____

Cooking Instructions:
_____
_____
_____
_____
_____
_____
_____
_____
_____
_____
_____

Thoughts and Notes:
_____
_____
_____
_____
_____

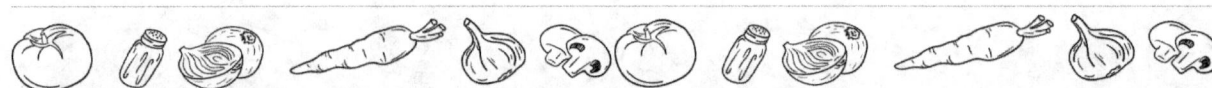

Recipe:

Rating: ☆☆☆☆☆ Difficulty: ☆☆☆☆☆ Prep Time: Cook Time:

Ingredients:

Cooking Instructions:

Thoughts and Notes:

Recipe: _____

Rating: ☆☆☆☆☆ Difficulty: ☆☆☆☆☆ Prep Time: _____ Cook Time: _____

Ingredients:
_____
_____
_____
_____
_____
_____
_____

Cooking Instructions: _____
_____
_____
_____
_____
_____
_____
_____
_____
_____
_____
_____
_____

Thoughts and Notes: _____
_____
_____
_____
_____
_____

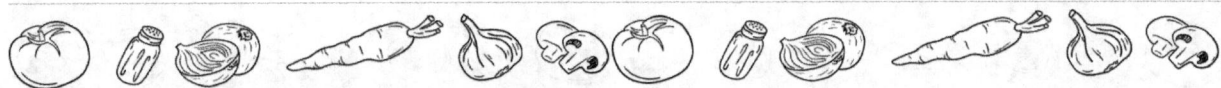

Recipe:

Rating: ☆☆☆☆☆ Difficulty: ☆☆☆☆☆ Prep Time: Cook Time:

Ingredients:

Cooking Instructions:

Thoughts and Notes:

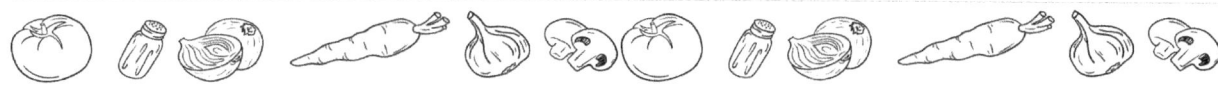

Recipe:

Rating: ☆☆☆☆☆ Difficulty: ☆☆☆☆☆ Prep Time: Cook Time:

Ingredients:

Cooking Instructions:

Thoughts and Notes:

Recipe:

Rating: ☆☆☆☆☆   Difficulty: ✿✿✿✿✿   Prep Time: Cook Time:

Ingredients:

Cooking Instructions:

Thoughts and Notes:

Recipe:

Rating: ☆☆☆☆☆ Difficulty: ✿✿✿✿✿ Prep Time: Cook Time:

Ingredients:

Cooking Instructions:

Thoughts and Notes:

Recipe:

Rating: ☆☆☆☆☆ Difficulty: ☆☆☆☆☆ Prep Time: Cook Time:

Ingredients:

Cooking Instructions:

Thoughts and Notes:

Recipe:

Rating: ☆☆☆☆☆ Difficulty: ☆☆☆☆☆ Prep Time: Cook Time:

Ingredients:
_____
_____
_____
_____
_____
_____

Cooking Instructions:
_____
_____
_____
_____
_____
_____
_____
_____
_____
_____
_____

Thoughts and Notes:
_____
_____
_____
_____
_____

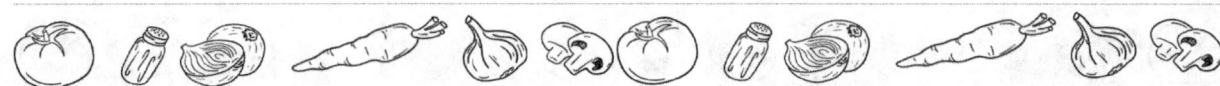

Recipe:

Rating: ☆☆☆☆☆ Difficulty: ☆☆☆☆☆ Prep Time: Cook Time:

Ingredients:

Cooking Instructions:

Thoughts and Notes:

Recipe:

Rating: ☆☆☆☆☆ Difficulty: ✿✿✿✿✿ Prep Time: Cook Time:

Ingredients:
___
___
___
___
___
___
___

Cooking Instructions:
___
___
___
___
___
___
___
___
___
___
___
___

Thoughts and Notes:
___
___
___
___
___
___

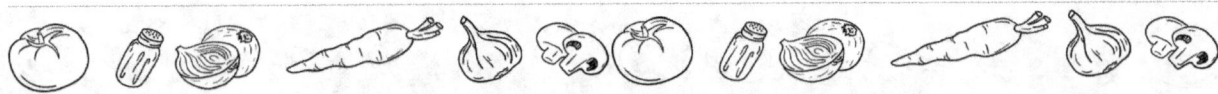

Recipe:

Rating: ☆☆☆☆☆ Difficulty: ☆☆☆☆☆ Prep Time: Cook Time:

Ingredients:

Cooking Instructions:

Thoughts and Notes:

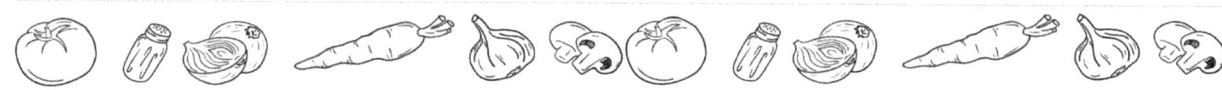

Recipe:

Rating: ☆☆☆☆☆ Difficulty: ☆☆☆☆☆ Prep Time: Cook Time:

Ingredients:

Cooking Instructions:

Thoughts and Notes:

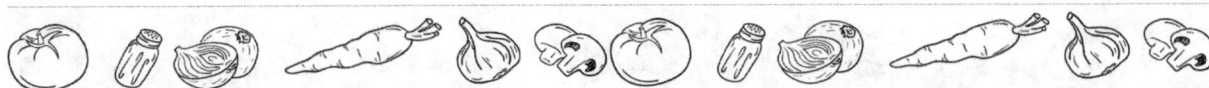

Recipe:

Rating: ☆☆☆☆☆ Difficulty: ☆☆☆☆☆ Prep Time: Cook Time:

Ingredients:

Cooking Instructions:

Thoughts and Notes:

Recipe:

Rating: ☆☆☆☆☆ Difficulty: ✿✿✿✿✿ Prep Time: Cook Time:

Ingredients:

Cooking Instructions:

Thoughts and Notes:

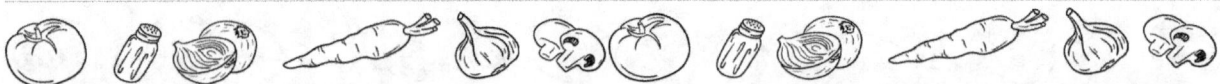

Recipe:

Rating: ☆☆☆☆☆ Difficulty: ☆☆☆☆☆ Prep Time: Cook Time:

Ingredients:

Cooking Instructions:

Thoughts and Notes:

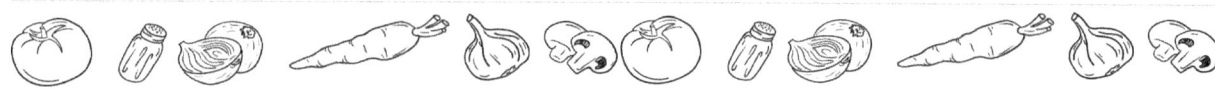

Recipe:

Rating: ☆☆☆☆☆ Difficulty: ☆☆☆☆☆ Prep Time: Cook Time:

Ingredients:

Cooking Instructions:

Thoughts and Notes:

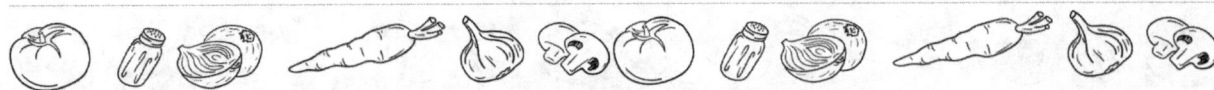

Recipe:

Rating: ☆☆☆☆☆ Difficulty: ☆☆☆☆☆ Prep Time: Cook Time:

Ingredients:

Cooking Instructions:

Thoughts and Notes:

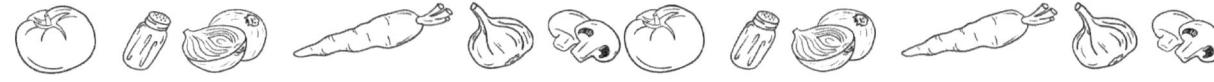

Recipe:

Rating: ☆☆☆☆☆ Difficulty: ✿✿✿✿✿ Prep Time: Cook Time:

Ingredients:

Cooking Instructions:

Thoughts and Notes:

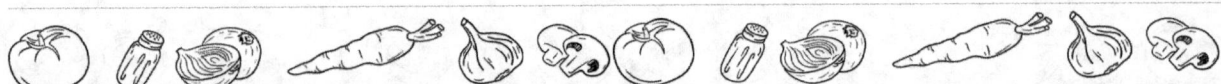

Recipe:

Rating: ☆☆☆☆☆ Difficulty: ☆☆☆☆☆ Prep Time: Cook Time:

Ingredients:

Cooking Instructions:

Thoughts and Notes:

Recipe:

Rating: ☆☆☆☆☆ Difficulty: ☆☆☆☆☆ Prep Time: Cook Time:

Ingredients:

Cooking Instructions:

Thoughts and Notes:

Recipe:

Rating: ☆☆☆☆☆ Difficulty: ☆☆☆☆☆ Prep Time: Cook Time:

Ingredients:

Cooking Instructions:

Thoughts and Notes:

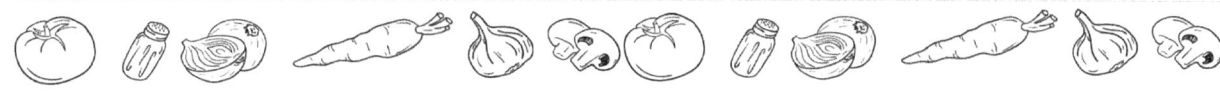

Recipe:

Rating: ☆☆☆☆☆ Difficulty: ☆☆☆☆☆ Prep Time: Cook Time:

Ingredients:

Cooking Instructions:

Thoughts and Notes:

Recipe:

Rating: ☆☆☆☆☆ Difficulty: ✿✿✿✿✿ Prep Time: Cook Time:

Ingredients:

Cooking Instructions:

Thoughts and Notes:

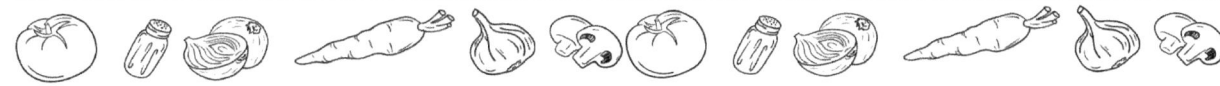

Recipe:

Rating: ☆☆☆☆☆ Difficulty: ☆☆☆☆☆ Prep Time: Cook Time:

Ingredients:
_____
_____
_____
_____
_____
_____

Cooking Instructions:
_____
_____
_____
_____
_____
_____
_____
_____
_____
_____
_____

Thoughts and Notes:
_____
_____
_____
_____
_____
_____

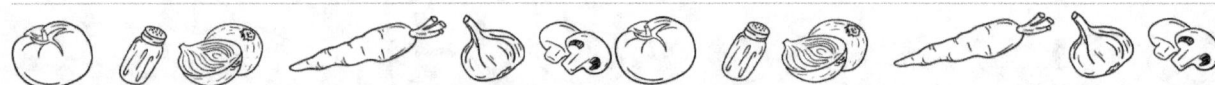

Recipe:

Rating: ☆☆☆☆☆ Difficulty: ☆☆☆☆☆ Prep Time: Cook Time:

Ingredients:

Cooking Instructions:

Thoughts and Notes:

Recipe:

Rating: ☆☆☆☆☆ Difficulty: ✿✿✿✿✿ Prep Time: Cook Time:

Ingredients:

Cooking Instructions:

Thoughts and Notes:

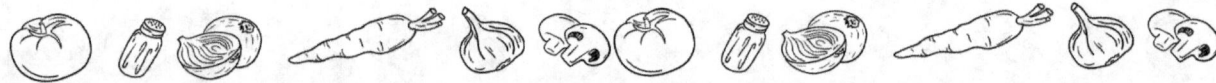

Recipe:

Rating: ☆☆☆☆☆ Difficulty: ☆☆☆☆☆ Prep Time: Cook Time:

Ingredients:

Cooking Instructions:

Thoughts and Notes:

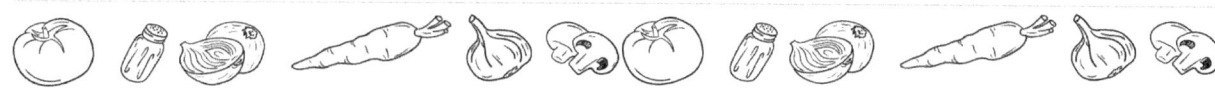

Recipe:

Rating: ☆☆☆☆☆ Difficulty: ☆☆☆☆☆ Prep Time:　　　　　Cook Time:

Ingredients:

Cooking Instructions:

Thoughts and Notes:

Recipe:

Rating: ☆☆☆☆☆ Difficulty: ☆☆☆☆☆ Prep Time: Cook Time:

Ingredients:

Cooking Instructions:

Thoughts and Notes:

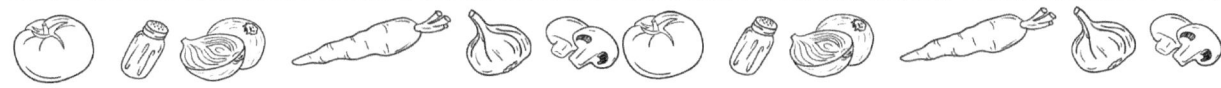

Recipe:

Rating: ☆☆☆☆ Difficulty: ✿✿✿✿ Prep Time: Cook Time:

Ingredients:
_____
_____
_____
_____
_____
_____

Cooking Instructions:
_____
_____
_____
_____
_____
_____
_____
_____
_____
_____
_____

Thoughts and Notes:
_____
_____
_____
_____
_____

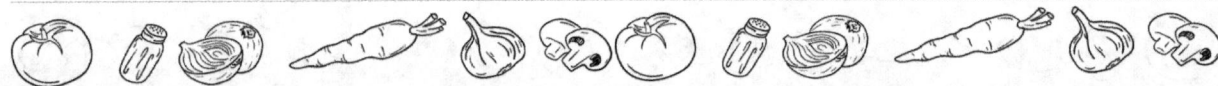

Recipe:

Rating: ☆☆☆☆☆ Difficulty: ☆☆☆☆☆ Prep Time: Cook Time:

Ingredients:

Cooking Instructions:

Thoughts and Notes:

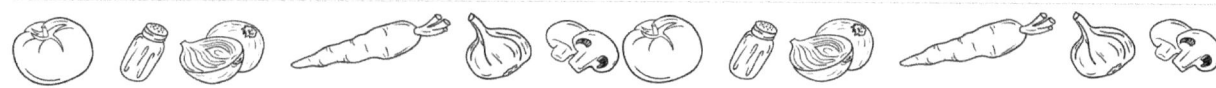

Recipe:

Rating: ☆☆☆☆☆ Difficulty: ✿✿✿✿✿ Prep Time: Cook Time:

Ingredients:

Cooking Instructions:

Thoughts and Notes:

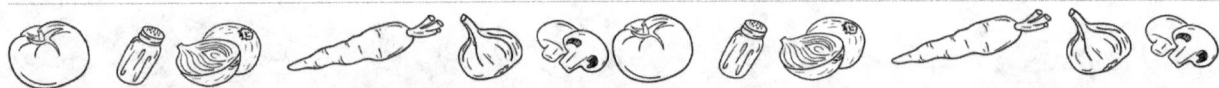

Recipe:

Rating: ☆☆☆☆☆ Difficulty: ☆☆☆☆☆ Prep Time: Cook Time:

Ingredients:

Cooking Instructions:

Thoughts and Notes:

Recipe:

Rating: ☆☆☆☆☆ Difficulty: ☆☆☆☆☆ Prep Time: Cook Time:

Ingredients:

Cooking Instructions:

Thoughts and Notes:

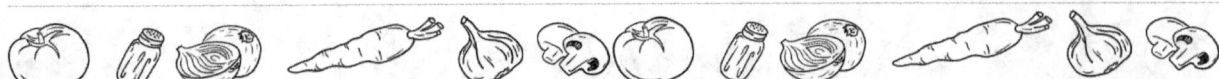

Recipe:

Rating: ☆☆☆☆☆ Difficulty: ☆☆☆☆☆ Prep Time: Cook Time:

Ingredients:

Cooking Instructions:

Thoughts and Notes:

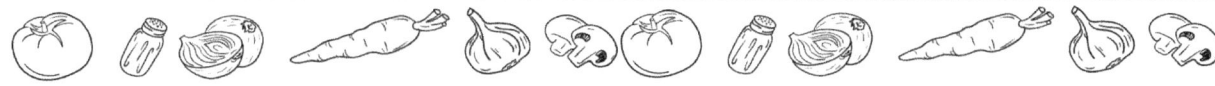

Recipe:

Rating: ☆☆☆☆☆ Difficulty: ☆☆☆☆☆ Prep Time: Cook Time:

Ingredients:

Cooking Instructions:

Thoughts and Notes:

Recipe:

Rating: ☆☆☆☆☆ Difficulty: ☆☆☆☆☆ Prep Time: Cook Time:

Ingredients:

Cooking Instructions:

Thoughts and Notes:

Recipe:

Rating: ☆☆☆☆☆ Difficulty: ☆☆☆☆☆ Prep Time: Cook Time:

Ingredients:
_____
_____
_____
_____
_____
_____

Cooking Instructions:
_____
_____
_____
_____
_____
_____
_____
_____
_____
_____
_____
_____

Thoughts and Notes:
_____
_____
_____
_____
_____

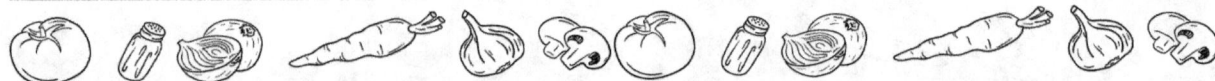

Recipe:

Rating: ☆☆☆☆☆ Difficulty: ✿✿✿✿✿ Prep Time: Cook Time:

Ingredients:

Cooking Instructions:

Thoughts and Notes:

Recipe:

Rating: ☆☆☆☆☆ Difficulty: ☆☆☆☆☆ Prep Time: Cook Time:

Ingredients:

_____
_____
_____
_____
_____
_____

Cooking Instructions:

_____
_____
_____
_____
_____
_____
_____
_____
_____
_____
_____

Thoughts and Notes:

_____
_____
_____
_____
_____

Recipe:

Rating: ☆☆☆☆☆ Difficulty: ☆☆☆☆☆ Prep Time: Cook Time:

Ingredients:

Cooking Instructions:

Thoughts and Notes:

Recipe:

Rating: ☆☆☆☆☆ Difficulty: ☆☆☆☆☆ Prep Time: Cook Time:

Ingredients:

Cooking Instructions:

Thoughts and Notes:

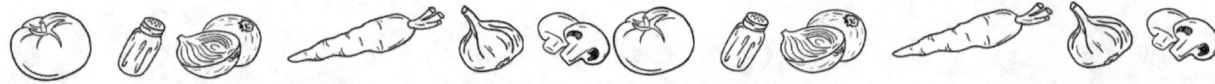

Recipe:

Rating: ☆☆☆☆☆ Difficulty: ☆☆☆☆☆ Prep Time: Cook Time:

Ingredients:

Cooking Instructions:

Thoughts and Notes:

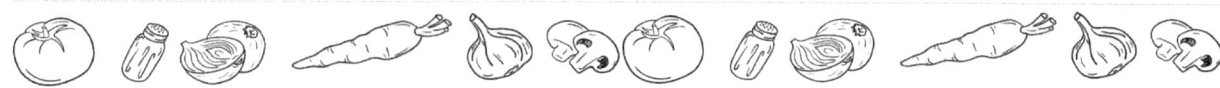

Recipe:

Rating: ☆☆☆☆☆ Difficulty: ☆☆☆☆☆ Prep Time: Cook Time:

Ingredients:

Cooking Instructions:

Thoughts and Notes:

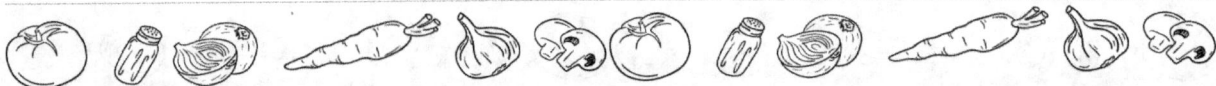

Recipe:

Rating: ☆☆☆☆☆ **Difficulty:** ☆☆☆☆☆ **Prep Time:**   **Cook Time:**

Ingredients:

Cooking Instructions:

Thoughts and Notes:

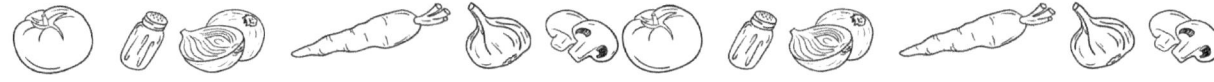

Recipe:

Rating: ☆☆☆☆ Difficulty: ✿✿✿✿ Prep Time: Cook Time:

Ingredients:

Cooking Instructions:

Thoughts and Notes:

Recipe:

Rating: ☆☆☆☆☆ Difficulty: ☆☆☆☆☆ Prep Time: Cook Time:

Ingredients:

Cooking Instructions:

Thoughts and Notes:

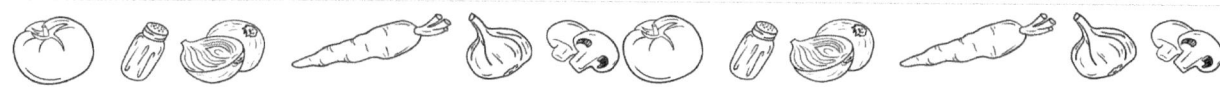

Recipe:

Rating: ☆☆☆☆☆ Difficulty: ☆☆☆☆☆ Prep Time: Cook Time:

Ingredients:

Cooking Instructions:

Thoughts and Notes:

Recipe:

Rating: ☆☆☆☆☆ Difficulty: ☆☆☆☆☆ Prep Time: Cook Time:

Ingredients:

Cooking Instructions:

Thoughts and Notes:

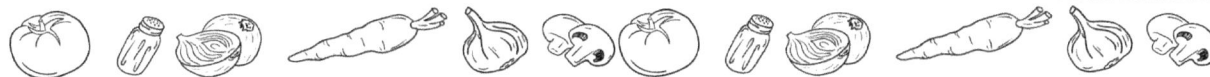

Recipe:

Rating: ☆☆☆☆☆ Difficulty: ✿✿✿✿✿ Prep Time: Cook Time:

Ingredients:

Cooking Instructions:

Thoughts and Notes:

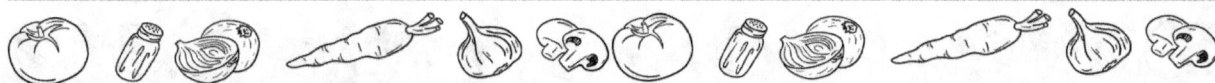

Recipe:

Rating: ☆☆☆☆☆ Difficulty: ✿✿✿✿✿ Prep Time: Cook Time:

Ingredients:

Cooking Instructions:

Thoughts and Notes:

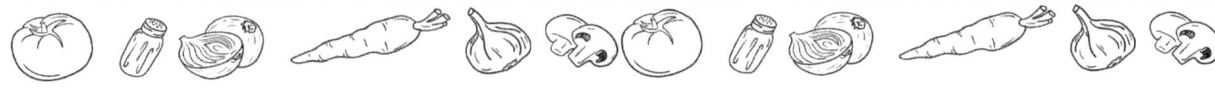

Recipe:

Rating: ☆☆☆☆ Difficulty: ✿✿✿✿ Prep Time: Cook Time:

Ingredients:
_____
_____
_____
_____
_____
_____

Cooking Instructions:
_____
_____
_____
_____
_____
_____
_____
_____
_____
_____
_____

Thoughts and Notes:
_____
_____
_____
_____
_____

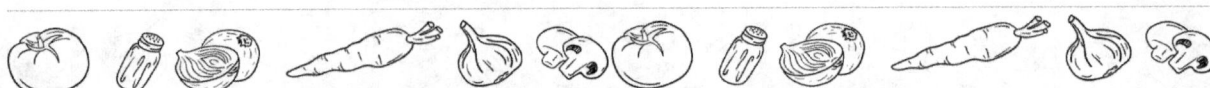

Recipe:

Rating: ☆☆☆☆☆ Difficulty: ☆☆☆☆☆ Prep Time: Cook Time:

Ingredients:

Cooking Instructions:

Thoughts and Notes:

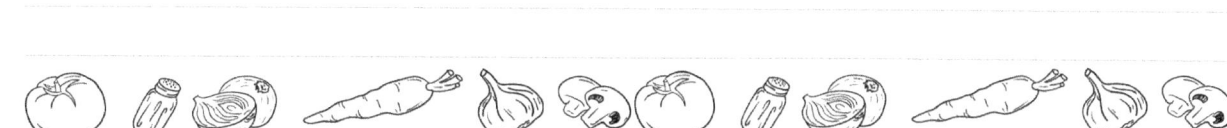

Recipe:

Rating: ☆☆☆☆　Difficulty: ✿✿✿✿　Prep Time:　　　　Cook Time:

Ingredients:

Cooking Instructions:

Thoughts and Notes:

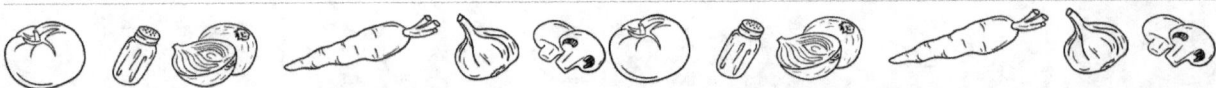

Recipe:

Rating: ☆☆☆☆☆ Difficulty: ☆☆☆☆☆ Prep Time: Cook Time:

Ingredients:

Cooking Instructions:

Thoughts and Notes:

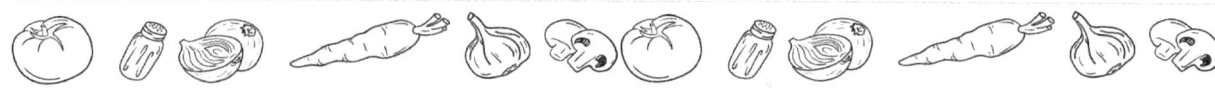

Recipe:

Rating: ☆☆☆☆☆ Difficulty: ☆☆☆☆☆ Prep Time: Cook Time:

Ingredients:

Cooking Instructions:

Thoughts and Notes:

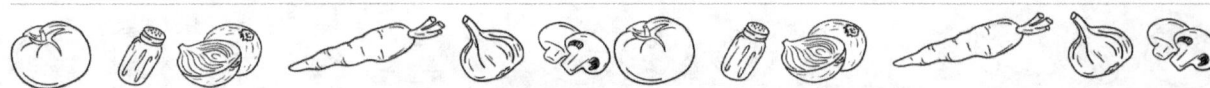

Recipe:

Rating: ☆☆☆☆☆ Difficulty: ☆☆☆☆☆ Prep Time: Cook Time:

Ingredients:

Cooking Instructions:

Thoughts and Notes:

Recipe:

Rating: ☆☆☆☆ Difficulty: ☆☆☆☆ Prep Time: Cook Time:

Ingredients:

Cooking Instructions:

Thoughts and Notes:

Recipe:

Rating: ☆☆☆☆☆ Difficulty: ☆☆☆☆☆ Prep Time: Cook Time:

Ingredients:

Cooking Instructions:

Thoughts and Notes:

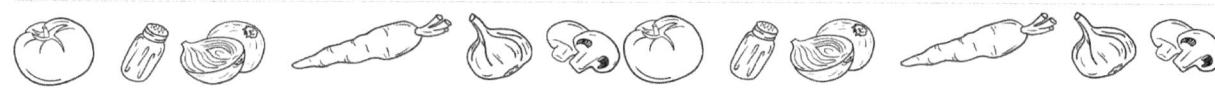

Recipe:

Rating: ☆☆☆☆☆ Difficulty: ☆☆☆☆☆ Prep Time: Cook Time:

Ingredients:

Cooking Instructions:

Thoughts and Notes:

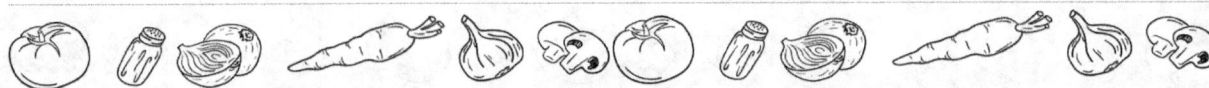

Recipe:

Rating: ☆☆☆☆☆ Difficulty: ☆☆☆☆☆ Prep Time: Cook Time:

Ingredients:

Cooking Instructions:

Thoughts and Notes:

Recipe:

Rating: ☆☆☆☆ Difficulty: ☆☆☆☆ Prep Time: Cook Time:

Ingredients:

Cooking Instructions:

Thoughts and Notes:

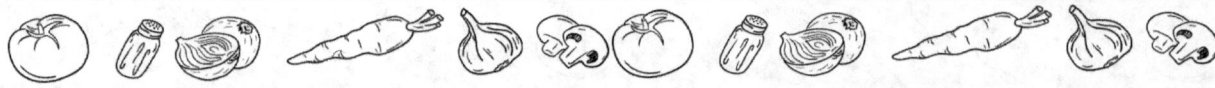

Recipe:

Rating: ☆☆☆☆☆ Difficulty: ☆☆☆☆☆ Prep Time: Cook Time:

Ingredients:

Cooking Instructions:

Thoughts and Notes:

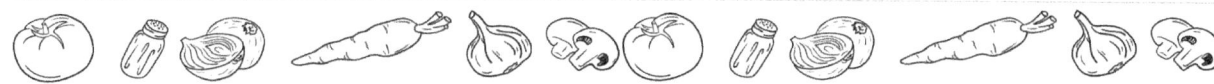

Recipe:

Rating: ☆☆☆☆☆ Difficulty: ☆☆☆☆☆ Prep Time: Cook Time:

Ingredients:

Cooking Instructions:

Thoughts and Notes:

Recipe:

Rating: ☆☆☆☆☆ Difficulty: ☆☆☆☆☆ Prep Time: Cook Time:

Ingredients:

Cooking Instructions:

Thoughts and Notes:

Recipe:

Rating: ☆☆☆☆☆ Difficulty: ✿✿✿✿✿ Prep Time: Cook Time:

Ingredients:

Cooking Instructions:

Thoughts and Notes:

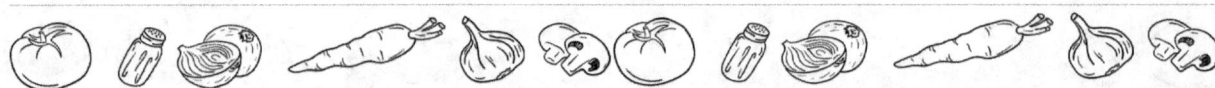

Recipe:

Rating: ☆☆☆☆☆ Difficulty: ☆☆☆☆☆ Prep Time: Cook Time:

Ingredients:

Cooking Instructions:

Thoughts and Notes:

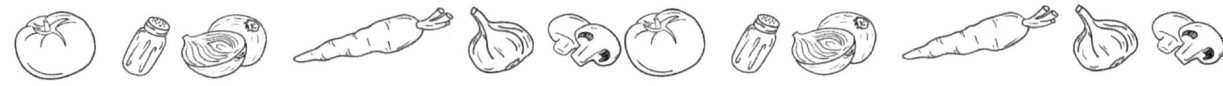

Recipe:

Rating: ☆☆☆☆☆ **Difficulty:** ☆☆☆☆☆ **Prep Time:**　　　　**Cook Time:**

Ingredients:

Cooking Instructions:

Thoughts and Notes:

Recipe:

Rating: ☆☆☆☆☆ Difficulty: ☆☆☆☆☆ Prep Time: Cook Time:

Ingredients:

Cooking Instructions:

Thoughts and Notes:

Recipe:

Rating: ☆☆☆☆☆   Difficulty: ✿✿✿✿✿   Prep Time: Cook Time:

Ingredients:

Cooking Instructions:

Thoughts and Notes:

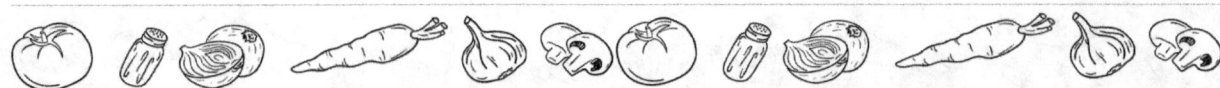

Recipe:

Rating: ☆☆☆☆☆ Difficulty: ☆☆☆☆☆ Prep Time: Cook Time:

Ingredients:

Cooking Instructions:

Thoughts and Notes:

Recipe:

Rating: ☆☆☆☆☆ Difficulty: ✿✿✿✿✿ Prep Time: Cook Time:

Ingredients:

Cooking Instructions:

Thoughts and Notes:

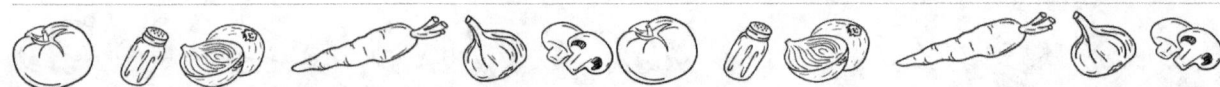

Recipe:

Rating: ☆☆☆☆☆ Difficulty: ☆☆☆☆☆ Prep Time: Cook Time:

Ingredients:

Cooking Instructions:

Thoughts and Notes:

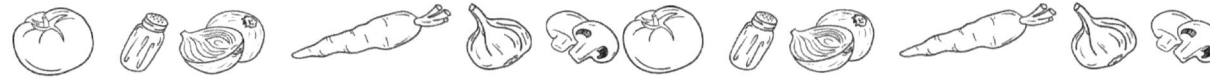

Recipe:

Rating: ☆☆☆☆ Difficulty: ✿✿✿✿ Prep Time: Cook Time:

Ingredients:

Cooking Instructions:

Thoughts and Notes:

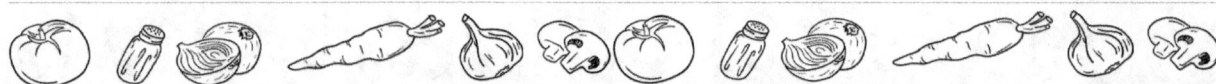

Recipe:

Rating: ☆☆☆☆☆ Difficulty: ☆☆☆☆☆ Prep Time:　　　　Cook Time:

Ingredients:

Cooking Instructions:

Thoughts and Notes:

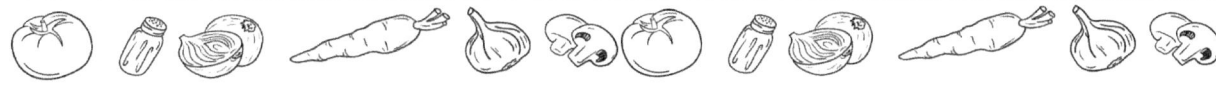

Recipe:

Rating: ☆☆☆☆☆   Difficulty: ☆☆☆☆☆   Prep Time: Cook Time:

Ingredients:

Cooking Instructions:

Thoughts and Notes:

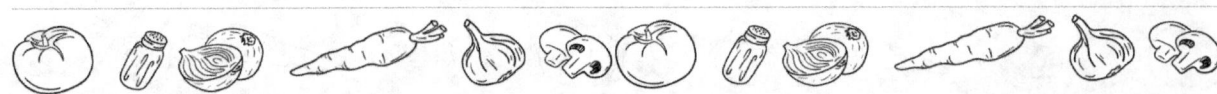

Recipe:

Rating: ☆☆☆☆☆ Difficulty: ☆☆☆☆☆ Prep Time: Cook Time:

Ingredients:

Cooking Instructions:

Thoughts and Notes:

Recipe:

Rating: ☆☆☆☆☆ Difficulty: ✿✿✿✿✿ Prep Time: Cook Time:

Ingredients:

Cooking Instructions:

Thoughts and Notes:

Recipe:

Rating: ☆☆☆☆☆ Difficulty: ☆☆☆☆☆ Prep Time: Cook Time:

Ingredients:

Cooking Instructions:

Thoughts and Notes:

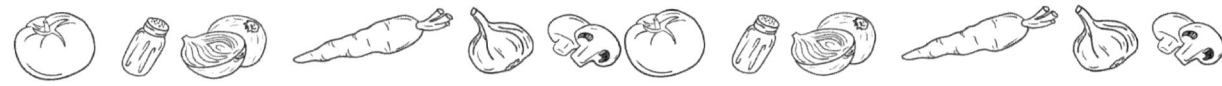

Recipe:

Rating: ☆☆☆☆☆ Difficulty: ☆☆☆☆☆ Prep Time: Cook Time:

Ingredients:

Cooking Instructions:

Thoughts and Notes:

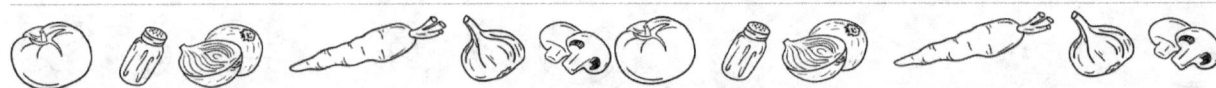

Recipe:

Rating: ☆☆☆☆☆ Difficulty: ☆☆☆☆☆ Prep Time: Cook Time:

Ingredients:

Cooking Instructions:

Thoughts and Notes:

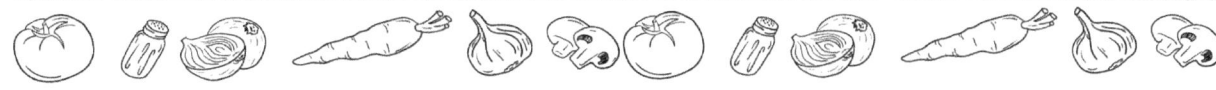

Recipe:

Rating: ☆☆☆☆☆ Difficulty: ❀❀❀❀❀ Prep Time: Cook Time:

Ingredients:

Cooking Instructions:

Thoughts and Notes:

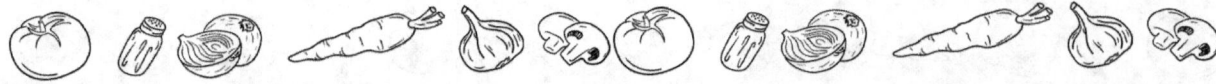

Recipe:

Rating: ☆☆☆☆☆ Difficulty: ☆☆☆☆☆ Prep Time: Cook Time:

Ingredients:

Cooking Instructions:

Thoughts and Notes:

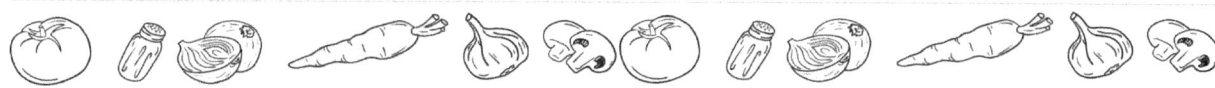

Recipe:

Rating: ☆☆☆☆☆ Difficulty: ☆☆☆☆☆ Prep Time: Cook Time:

Ingredients:

Cooking Instructions:

Thoughts and Notes:

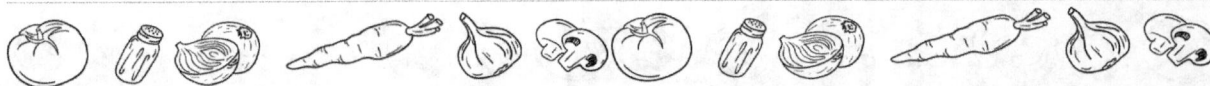

Recipe:

Rating: ☆☆☆☆☆ Difficulty: ☆☆☆☆☆ Prep Time: Cook Time:

Ingredients:

Cooking Instructions:

Thoughts and Notes:

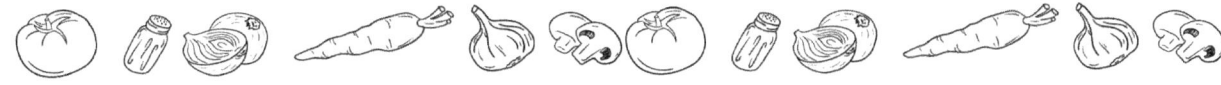

Recipe:

Rating: ☆☆☆☆☆ Difficulty: ✿✿✿✿✿ Prep Time: Cook Time:

Ingredients:

Cooking Instructions:

Thoughts and Notes:

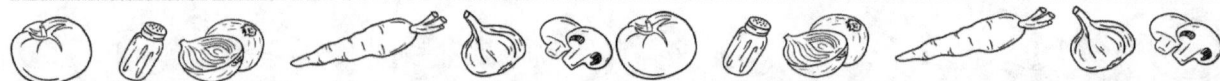

Recipe:

Rating: ☆☆☆☆☆ Difficulty: ☆☆☆☆☆ Prep Time: Cook Time:

Ingredients:

Cooking Instructions:

Thoughts and Notes:

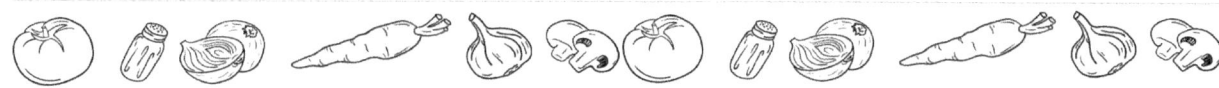

Recipe:

Rating: ☆☆☆☆☆ **Difficulty:** ☆☆☆☆☆ **Prep Time:** **Cook Time:**

Ingredients:

Cooking Instructions:

Thoughts and Notes:

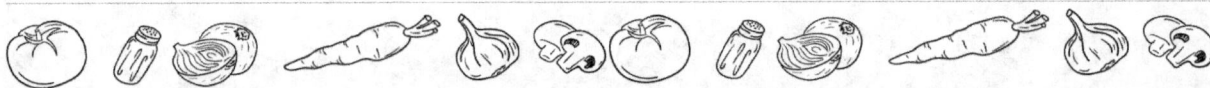

Recipe:

Rating: ☆☆☆☆☆ Difficulty: ☆☆☆☆☆ Prep Time: Cook Time:

Ingredients:

Cooking Instructions:

Thoughts and Notes:

Recipe:

Rating: ☆☆☆☆☆ Difficulty: ☆☆☆☆☆ Prep Time: Cook Time:

Ingredients:

Cooking Instructions:

Thoughts and Notes:

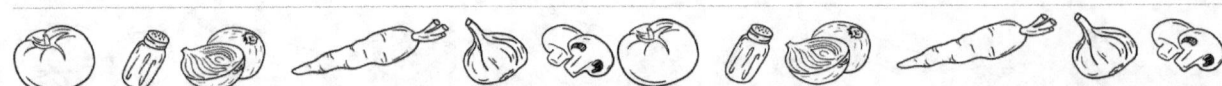

Recipe:

Rating: ☆☆☆☆☆ Difficulty: ☆☆☆☆☆ Prep Time: Cook Time:

Ingredients:

Cooking Instructions:

Thoughts and Notes:

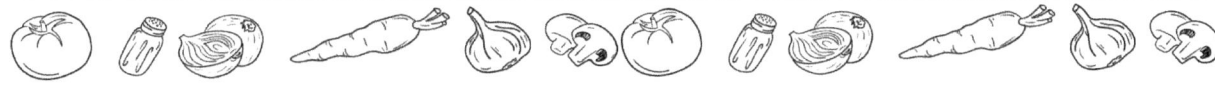

Recipe:

Rating: ☆☆☆☆☆ Difficulty: ☆☆☆☆☆ Prep Time: Cook Time:

Ingredients:

Cooking Instructions:

Thoughts and Notes:

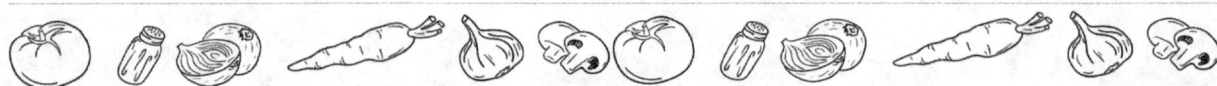

Recipe:

Rating: ☆☆☆☆☆ Difficulty: ☆☆☆☆☆ Prep Time: Cook Time:

Ingredients:

Cooking Instructions:

Thoughts and Notes:

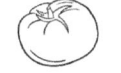 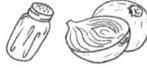 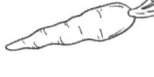 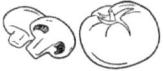   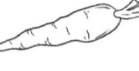 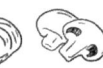

Recipe:

Rating: ☆☆☆☆☆ Difficulty: ✿✿✿✿✿ Prep Time: Cook Time:

Ingredients:

Cooking Instructions:

Thoughts and Notes:

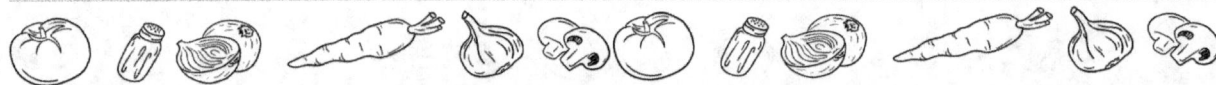

Recipe:

Rating: ☆☆☆☆☆ Difficulty: ☆☆☆☆☆ Prep Time: Cook Time:

Ingredients:

Cooking Instructions:

Thoughts and Notes:

Recipe:

Rating: ☆☆☆☆☆ Difficulty: ❀❀❀❀❀ Prep Time: Cook Time:

Ingredients:

Cooking Instructions:

Thoughts and Notes:

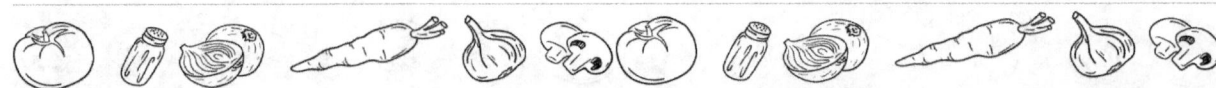

Recipe:

Rating: ☆☆☆☆☆ Difficulty: ☆☆☆☆☆ Prep Time: Cook Time:

Ingredients:

Cooking Instructions:

Thoughts and Notes:

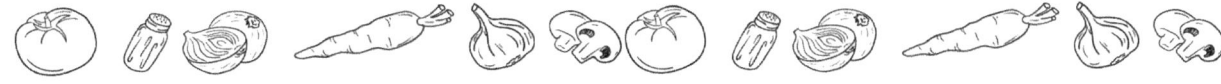

Recipe: _____

Rating: ☆☆☆☆☆ Difficulty: ❀❀❀❀❀ Prep Time: _____ Cook Time: _____

Ingredients:
_____
_____
_____
_____
_____
_____
_____

Cooking Instructions:
_____
_____
_____
_____
_____
_____
_____
_____
_____
_____
_____
_____

Thoughts and Notes:
_____
_____
_____
_____
_____

Recipe:

Rating: ☆☆☆☆☆ Difficulty: ☆☆☆☆☆ Prep Time: Cook Time:

Ingredients:

Cooking Instructions:

Thoughts and Notes:

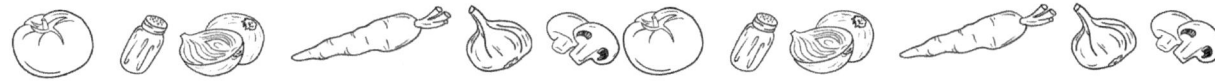

Recipe:

Rating: ☆☆☆☆☆ Difficulty: ☆☆☆☆☆ Prep Time: Cook Time:

Ingredients:

Cooking Instructions:

Thoughts and Notes:

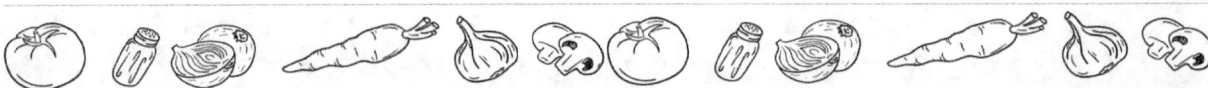

Recipe:

Rating: ☆☆☆☆☆ **Difficulty:** ☆☆☆☆☆ **Prep Time:**   **Cook Time:**

Ingredients:

Cooking Instructions:

Thoughts and Notes:

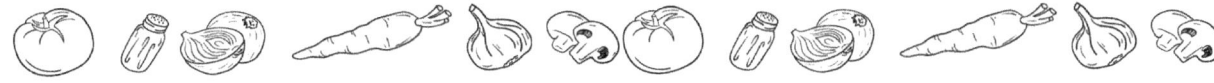

Recipe:

Rating: ☆☆☆☆☆ Difficulty: ✿✿✿✿✿ Prep Time: Cook Time:

Ingredients:
_____
_____
_____
_____
_____
_____

Cooking Instructions:
_____
_____
_____
_____
_____
_____
_____
_____
_____
_____

Thoughts and Notes:
_____
_____
_____
_____
_____

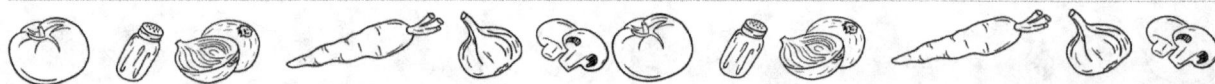

Recipe:

Rating: ☆☆☆☆☆ Difficulty: ☆☆☆☆☆ Prep Time:　　　　　Cook Time:

Ingredients:

Cooking Instructions:

Thoughts and Notes:

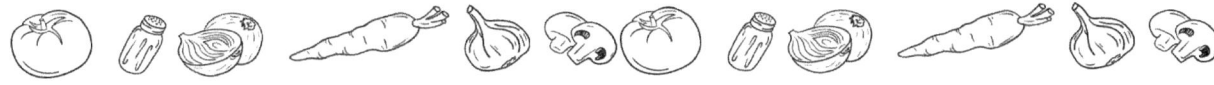

Recipe:

Rating: ☆☆☆☆☆ Difficulty: ☆☆☆☆☆ Prep Time: Cook Time:

Ingredients:

Cooking Instructions:

Thoughts and Notes:

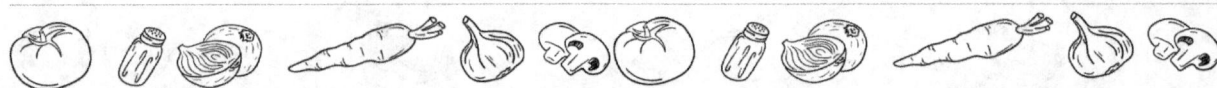

Recipe:

Rating: ☆☆☆☆☆ Difficulty: ☆☆☆☆☆ Prep Time: Cook Time:

Ingredients:

Cooking Instructions:

Thoughts and Notes:

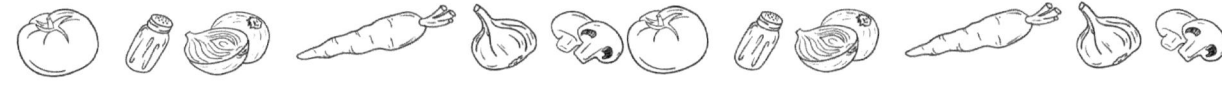

Recipe:

Rating: ☆☆☆☆ Difficulty: ☆☆☆☆ Prep Time: Cook Time:

Ingredients:

Cooking Instructions:

Thoughts and Notes:

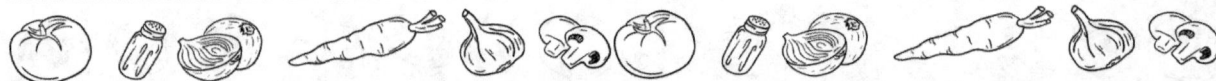

Recipe:

Rating: ☆☆☆☆☆ Difficulty: ☆☆☆☆☆ Prep Time: Cook Time:

Ingredients:

Cooking Instructions:

Thoughts and Notes:

Recipe:

Rating: ☆☆☆☆☆ Difficulty: ☆☆☆☆☆ Prep Time: Cook Time:

Ingredients:

Cooking Instructions:

Thoughts and Notes:

Recipe:

Rating: ☆☆☆☆☆ Difficulty: ☆☆☆☆☆ Prep Time: Cook Time:

Ingredients:

Cooking Instructions:

Thoughts and Notes:

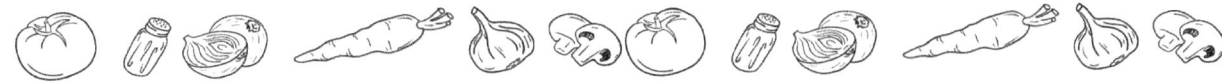

Recipe:

Rating: ☆☆☆☆ Difficulty: ✿✿✿✿ Prep Time: Cook Time:

Ingredients:

Cooking Instructions:

Thoughts and Notes:

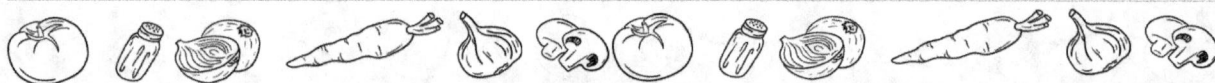

Recipe:

Rating: ☆☆☆☆☆ Difficulty: ☆☆☆☆☆ Prep Time: Cook Time:

Ingredients:

Cooking Instructions:

Thoughts and Notes:

Recipe:

Rating: ☆☆☆☆☆   Difficulty: ☆☆☆☆☆   Prep Time: Cook Time:

Ingredients:

Cooking Instructions:

Thoughts and Notes:

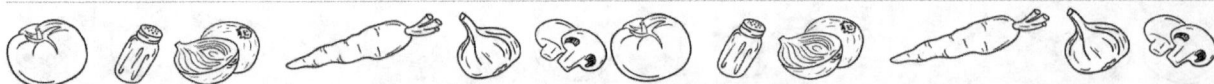

Recipe:

Rating: ☆☆☆☆☆ Difficulty: ☆☆☆☆☆ Prep Time: Cook Time:

Ingredients:

Cooking Instructions:

Thoughts and Notes:

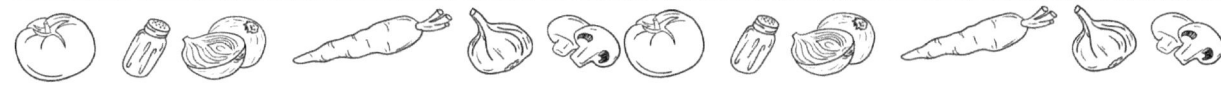

Recipe:

Rating: ☆☆☆☆ Difficulty: ✿✿✿✿ Prep Time: Cook Time:

Ingredients:
_____
_____
_____
_____
_____
_____

Cooking Instructions:
_____
_____
_____
_____
_____
_____
_____
_____
_____
_____
_____

Thoughts and Notes:
_____
_____
_____
_____
_____

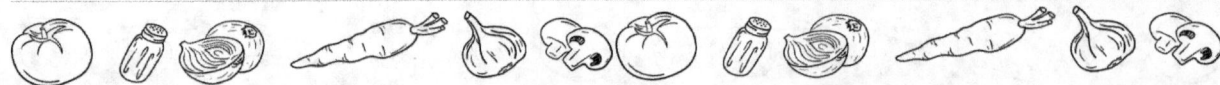

Recipe:

Rating: ☆☆☆☆☆ Difficulty: ☆☆☆☆☆ Prep Time: Cook Time:

Ingredients:

Cooking Instructions:

Thoughts and Notes:

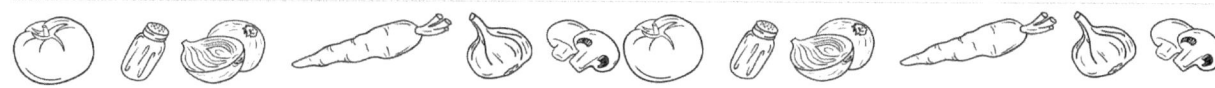

Recipe:

Rating: ☆☆☆☆☆ Difficulty: ☆☆☆☆☆ Prep Time: Cook Time:

Ingredients:

Cooking Instructions:

Thoughts and Notes:

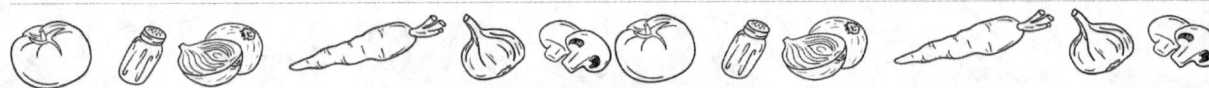

Recipe:

Rating: ☆☆☆☆☆ **Difficulty:** ☆☆☆☆☆ **Prep Time:**   **Cook Time:**

Ingredients:

Cooking Instructions:

Thoughts and Notes:

Recipe:

Rating: ☆☆☆☆☆ Difficulty: ✿✿✿✿✿ Prep Time: Cook Time:

Ingredients:

Cooking Instructions:

Thoughts and Notes:

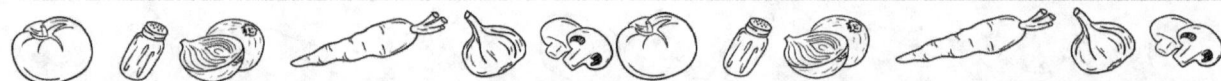

Recipe:

Rating: ☆☆☆☆☆ Difficulty: ☆☆☆☆☆ Prep Time: Cook Time:

Ingredients:

Cooking Instructions:

Thoughts and Notes:

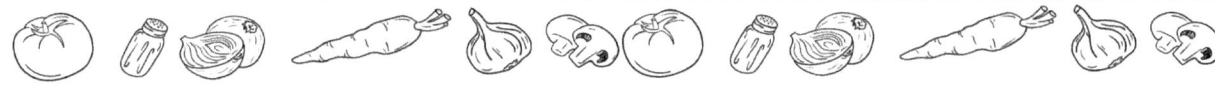

Recipe:

Rating: ☆☆☆☆☆ Difficulty: ✿✿✿✿✿ Prep Time: Cook Time:

Ingredients:

Cooking Instructions:

Thoughts and Notes:

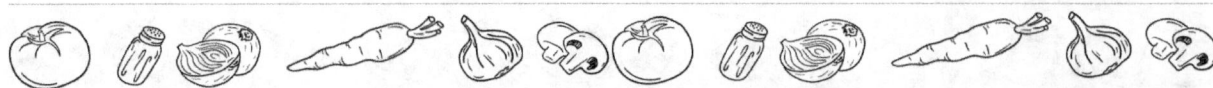

Recipe:

Rating: ☆☆☆☆☆ Difficulty: ☆☆☆☆☆ Prep Time: Cook Time:

Ingredients:

Cooking Instructions:

Thoughts and Notes:

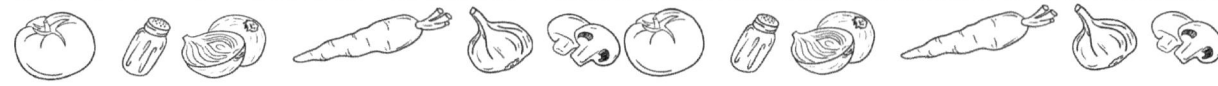

Recipe:

Rating: ☆☆☆☆☆ Difficulty: ✿✿✿✿✿ Prep Time: Cook Time:

Ingredients:

Cooking Instructions:

Thoughts and Notes:

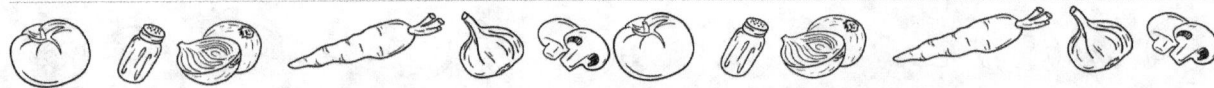

Recipe:

Rating: ☆☆☆☆☆ Difficulty: ☆☆☆☆☆ Prep Time: Cook Time:

Ingredients:

Cooking Instructions:

Thoughts and Notes:

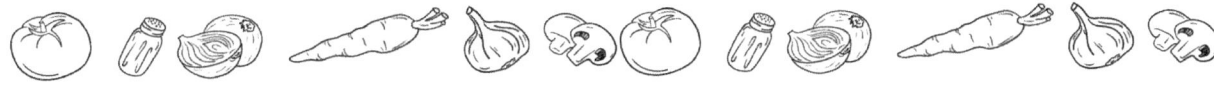

Recipe:

Rating: ☆☆☆☆☆ Difficulty: ☆☆☆☆☆ Prep Time: Cook Time:

Ingredients:
_____
_____
_____
_____
_____
_____

Cooking Instructions:
_____
_____
_____
_____
_____
_____
_____
_____
_____
_____
_____

Thoughts and Notes:
_____
_____
_____
_____
_____

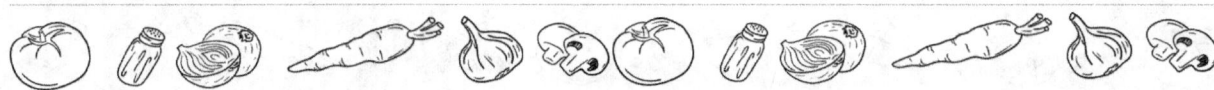

Recipe:

Rating: ☆☆☆☆☆ Difficulty: ☆☆☆☆☆ Prep Time: Cook Time:

Ingredients:

Cooking Instructions:

Thoughts and Notes:

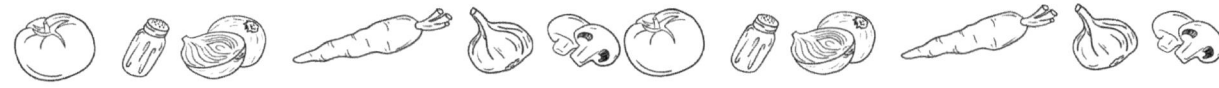

Recipe:

Rating: ☆☆☆☆☆ Difficulty: ☆☆☆☆☆ Prep Time: Cook Time:

Ingredients:

Cooking Instructions:

Thoughts and Notes:

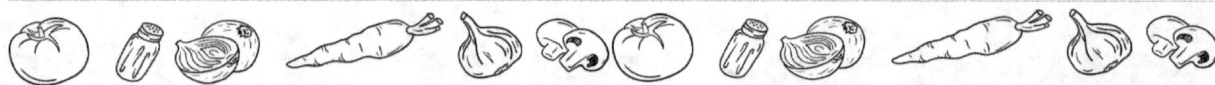

Recipe:

Rating: ☆☆☆☆☆ Difficulty: ☆☆☆☆☆ Prep Time: Cook Time:

Ingredients:

Cooking Instructions:

Thoughts and Notes:

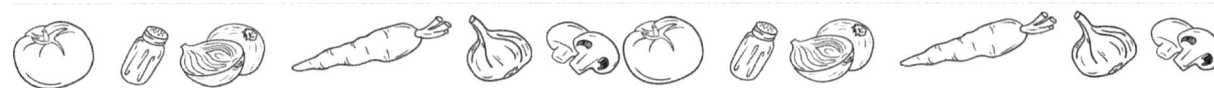

Recipe:

Rating: ☆☆☆☆☆ **Difficulty:** ☆☆☆☆☆ **Prep Time:**   **Cook Time:**

Ingredients:

Cooking Instructions:

Thoughts and Notes:

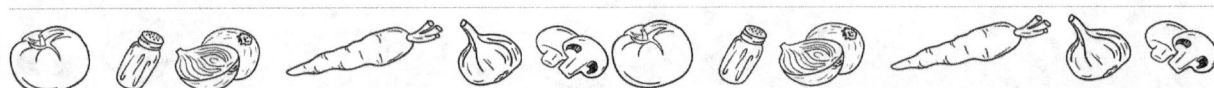

Recipe:

Rating: ☆☆☆☆☆ Difficulty: ☆☆☆☆☆ Prep Time: Cook Time:

Ingredients:

Cooking Instructions:

Thoughts and Notes:

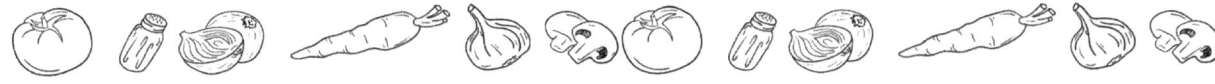

Recipe:

Rating: ☆☆☆☆ Difficulty: ✿✿✿✿ Prep Time: Cook Time:

Ingredients:

Cooking Instructions:

Thoughts and Notes:

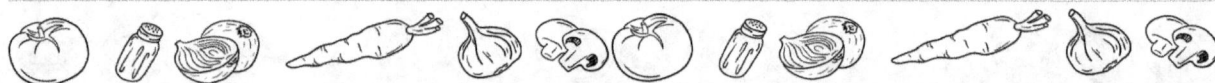

Recipe:

Rating: ☆☆☆☆☆   Difficulty: ☆☆☆☆☆   Prep Time: Cook Time:

Ingredients:

Cooking Instructions:

Thoughts and Notes:

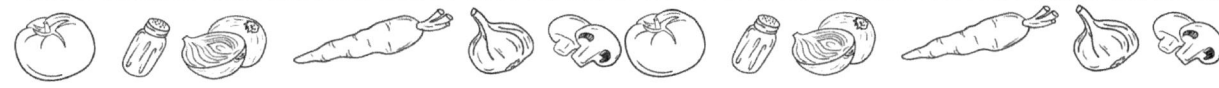

Recipe:

Rating: ☆☆☆☆☆ **Difficulty:** ☆☆☆☆☆ **Prep Time:**   **Cook Time:**

Ingredients:

Cooking Instructions:

Thoughts and Notes:

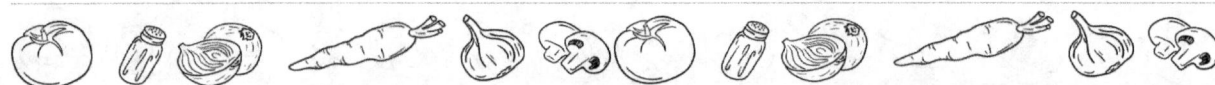

Recipe:

Rating: ☆☆☆☆☆ Difficulty: ☆☆☆☆☆ Prep Time: Cook Time:

Ingredients:

Cooking Instructions:

Thoughts and Notes:

Recipe:

Rating: ☆☆☆☆☆ Difficulty: ☆☆☆☆☆ Prep Time: Cook Time:

Ingredients:

Cooking Instructions:

Thoughts and Notes:

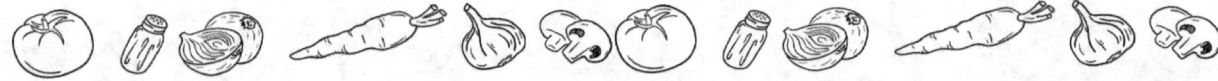

Recipe:

Rating: ☆☆☆☆☆ **Difficulty:** ☆☆☆☆☆ **Prep Time:**   **Cook Time:**

Ingredients:

Cooking Instructions:

Thoughts and Notes:

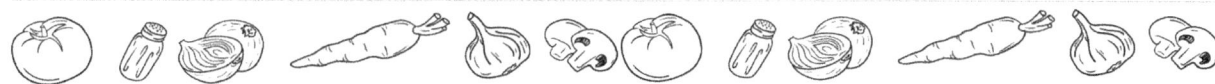

Recipe:

Rating: ☆☆☆☆☆ **Difficulty:** ☆☆☆☆☆ **Prep Time:** **Cook Time:**

Ingredients:

Cooking Instructions:

Thoughts and Notes:

Recipe:

Rating: ☆☆☆☆☆ Difficulty: ☆☆☆☆☆ Prep Time: Cook Time:

Ingredients:

Cooking Instructions:

Thoughts and Notes:

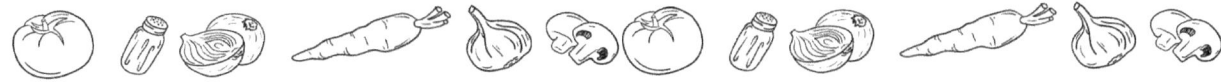

Recipe:

Rating: ☆☆☆☆☆ Difficulty: ☆☆☆☆☆ Prep Time: Cook Time:

Ingredients:

Cooking Instructions:

Thoughts and Notes:

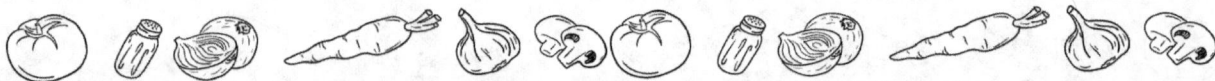

Recipe:

Rating: ☆☆☆☆☆ Difficulty: ☆☆☆☆☆ Prep Time: Cook Time:

Ingredients:

Cooking Instructions:

Thoughts and Notes:

Recipe:

Rating: ☆☆☆☆☆ Difficulty: ☆☆☆☆☆ Prep Time: _____ Cook Time: _____

Ingredients:
_____
_____
_____
_____
_____
_____
_____

Cooking Instructions:
_____
_____
_____
_____
_____
_____
_____
_____
_____
_____
_____
_____

Thoughts and Notes:
_____
_____
_____
_____
_____
_____

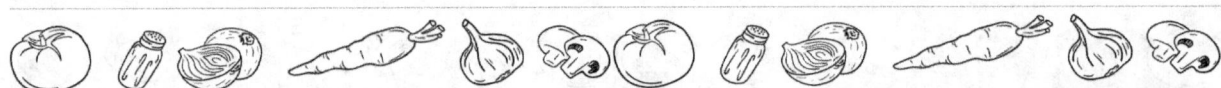

Recipe:

Rating: ☆☆☆☆☆ Difficulty: ☆☆☆☆☆ Prep Time: Cook Time:

Ingredients:

Cooking Instructions:

Thoughts and Notes:

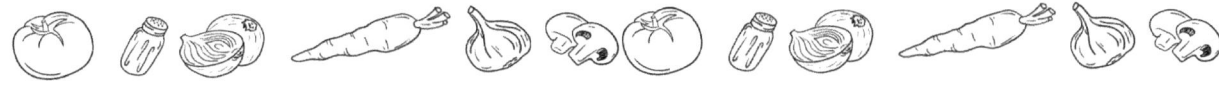

Recipe:

Rating: ☆☆☆☆☆ Difficulty: ☆☆☆☆☆ Prep Time: Cook Time:

Ingredients:

Cooking Instructions:

Thoughts and Notes:

Recipe:

Rating: ☆☆☆☆☆ Difficulty: ☆☆☆☆☆ Prep Time: Cook Time:

Ingredients:

Cooking Instructions:

Thoughts and Notes:

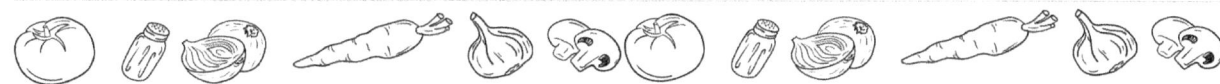

Recipe:

Rating: ☆☆☆☆☆ Difficulty: ☆☆☆☆☆ Prep Time:　　　　　Cook Time:

Ingredients:

Cooking Instructions:

Thoughts and Notes:

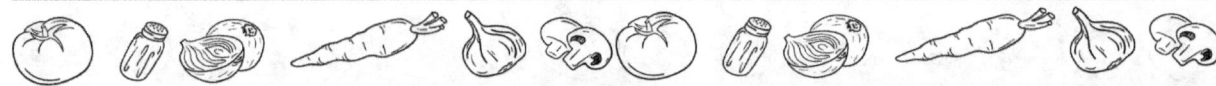

Recipe:

Rating: ☆☆☆☆☆ Difficulty: ☆☆☆☆☆ Prep Time: Cook Time:

Ingredients:

Cooking Instructions:

Thoughts and Notes:

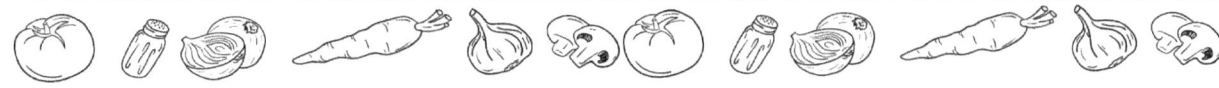

Recipe:

Rating: ☆☆☆☆☆ Difficulty: ☆☆☆☆☆ Prep Time: Cook Time:

Ingredients:
_____
_____
_____
_____
_____
_____
_____
_____

Cooking Instructions:
_____
_____
_____
_____
_____
_____
_____
_____
_____
_____
_____
_____
_____

Thoughts and Notes:
_____
_____
_____
_____
_____
_____

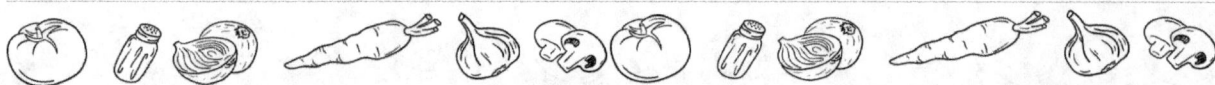

Recipe:

Rating: ☆☆☆☆☆ Difficulty: ✿✿✿✿✿ Prep Time: Cook Time:

Ingredients:

Cooking Instructions:

Thoughts and Notes:

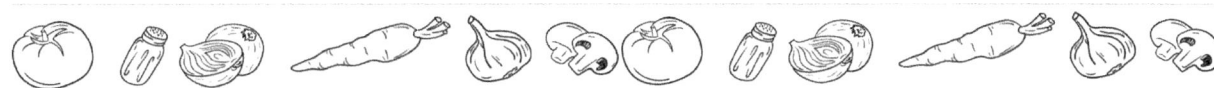

Recipe:

Rating: ☆☆☆☆☆ Difficulty: ☆☆☆☆☆ Prep Time: Cook Time:

Ingredients:

Cooking Instructions:

Thoughts and Notes:

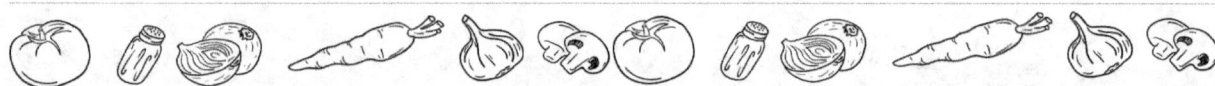